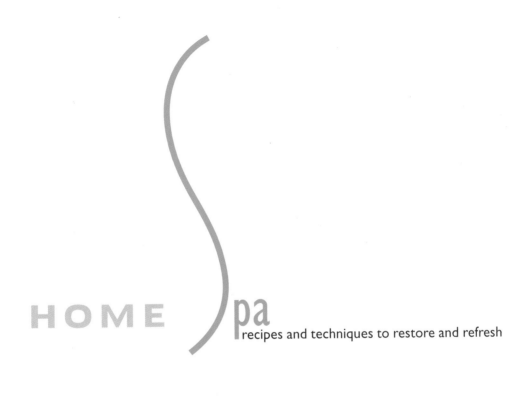

HOME Spa

recipes and techniques to restore and refresh

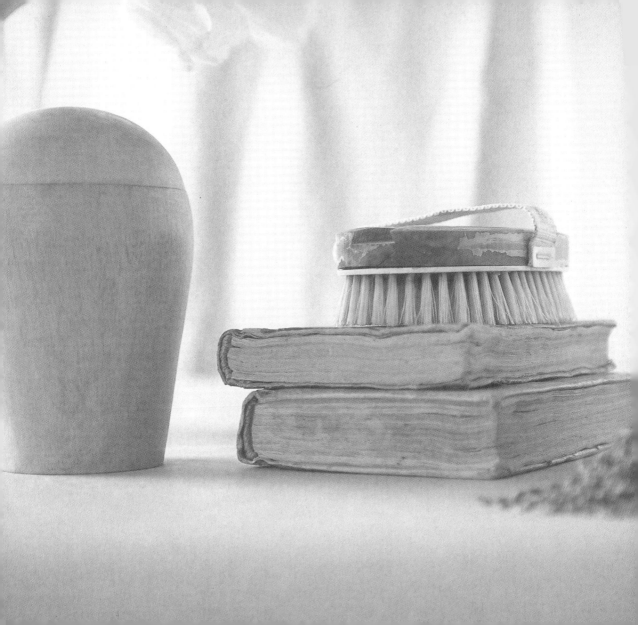

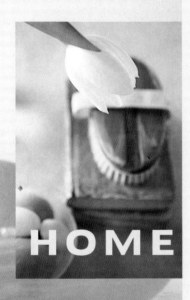

HOME Spa

recipes and techniques to restore and refresh

by Manine Rosa Golden

Principal photography by Marsha Burns

Abbeville Press   Publishers
New York   London   Paris

Concept: Jesianne Asagi

Design: Noreen Ryan

Art Direction: Manine Rosa Golden

Editing: Marie Weiler and Meredith Wolf with assistance by Sharon Rose Vonasch

Produced by Marquand Books, Inc.

The text of this book was set in Doric Bold, Gill Sans, and Duchamp.

Printed in Hong Kong.

First edition
10 9 8 7 6 5 4 3 2 1

Library of Congress Cataloging-in-Publication Data
Golden, Manine Rosa, 1969–
    Home spa : recipes and techniques to restore and refresh / by Manine Rosa Golden ; principal photography by Marsha Burns.
        p.   cm.
    Includes index.
    ISBN 0-7892-0346-4
    1. Beauty, Personal. 2. Women—Health and hygiene. 3. Herbal cosmetics. I. Title.
    RA778.G684   1997
    646.7'042—dc21   96-37074

The recipes and techniques in Home Spa *are intended for cosmetic and relaxation use only and are not meant to replace diagnosis and treatment by a qualified medical practitioner. The psychological and therapeutic benefits of the essential oils discussed in this book are based on traditional knowledge and experience. All recommendations herein contained have been tested to be safe. However, since some people have more sensitive skin than others and since the user's actual recipe preparation is beyond the control of the author or publisher, no express or implied guarantee or warranty as to the effects of their use is given by the author or publisher. Author and publisher accept no liability with regard to use of the recipes and techniques contained in this book. Make sure to test your skin for allergic reactions to any mixtures in this book 24 hours before applying treatment.*

Essential oils should not be taken internally nor should they be applied to the skin in pure concentration. If you are pregnant or have a medical condition, consult both a qualified aromatherapist and a doctor before using essential oils.

CONTENTS

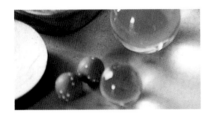

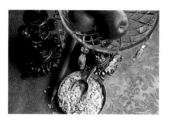

"I think my skin is turning blue."

"What?!" says your friend.

"My skin is taking on the color of my computer screen," you say. "And if I have to deal with another rush hour commute, I'll definitely turn blue in the face."

"You need a break," says your friend. "You are overworked and underpampered."

Stress builds up in our lives, manifesting itself in many ways. Is your skin breaking out? Do you have a hard time falling asleep? These problems could be stress related. Studies have shown that stress weakens the immune system, leaving the whole body more susceptible to illness. Healthy, balanced living begins with giving the right kind of attention to your body and mind. While most of us know this to be true, the fact is buried somewhere beneath the schedules and pressures of our daily lives. We are consumed with our jobs, engulfed by our commitments, and attacked daily by sun, wind, and environmental pollution—our hectic routines clog both our spirits and our pores.

Now you can take matters into your own hands. *Home Spa* is your secret weapon against the drudgery of routine and the pressures of environment, offering a variety of ways for you to relax and to look and feel better. You can

INTRODUCTION

treat yourself to many of the benefits of a day spa without leaving your home—and without the expense or time commitment of professional treatments. Using natural, readily available ingredients that you may already have in your refrigerator or cupboard, *Home Spa* provides easy recipes and techniques to revitalize yourself—from softening skin and relaxing tired muscles to removing toxins and improving circulation. Manufactured beauty products contain many ingredients you don't need, such as alcohol, chemicals, and artificial colorings, which often contribute more to dryness, itching, and rashes than to the care of your skin. Making your own spa products is not only more fun and less expensive than buying manufactured products, it puts you in control of what you put on your body.

While nothing can take the place of a weekend spa retreat or a holiday in the Caribbean, we'll show you inexpensive, easy ways to re-create professional spa techniques and a soothing environment in your own home. Whether you have half an hour or two days, *Home Spa* gives you the recipes and techniques to step out of your hectic routine and experience a renewed sense of calm and improved physical well-being.

Here are ways for you to pamper yourself from head to toe whenever you need it most—regardless of time or money. Taking the time to indulge yourself will ease life's pressures, clear your mind, and leave you feeling fresher and more capable of handling whatever comes your way.

It's time you put yourself at the top of your list of "things to take care of."

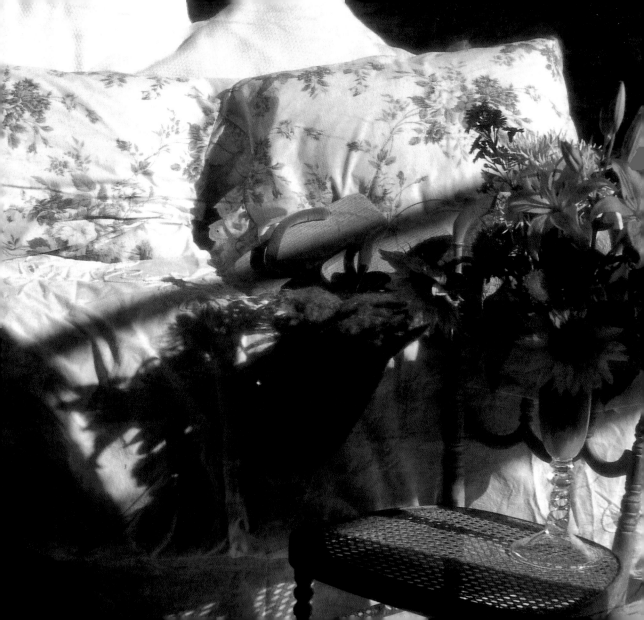

ENVIRONMENT

All the rubs and scrubs in the world cannot help cleanse your body or clear your mind if you're distracted by a ringing phone, tomorrow morning's meeting, or a pile of laundry. Before you begin any of your home spa treatments, consider the mood you are in vis-à-vis the mood you want to be in. Once you've given yourself full permission to set aside time just for you, don't allow anything else to intrude on your time. Turn off the ringer on the phone, forget about tomorrow's meeting for now, and create a soothing environment in your home. Fill a basket with natural sponges and loofah for your bath, and stack an assortment of thick towels in a variety of colors by the tub. Place candles and lanterns throughout the house to replace harsh electric lighting. The environment you create during your home spa pampering—whether it's a five-minute facial or a two-hour body scrub and wrap—affects how deeply you absorb the relaxing, restorative, healing qualities of the treatment.

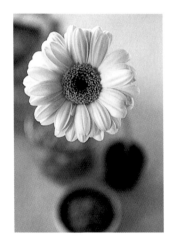

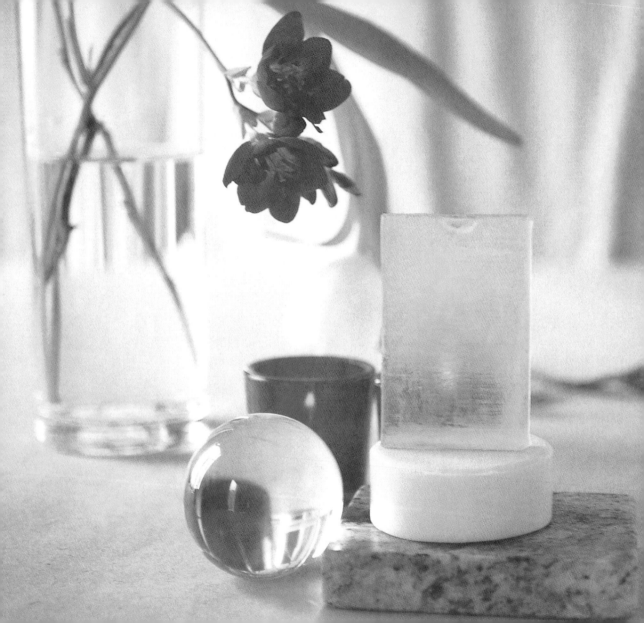

PLANTS

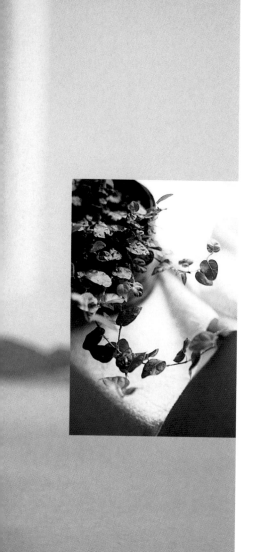

Surrounding yourself with plants and flowers is a simple way to create a warm, welcoming, and soothing ambience. Houseplants remove pollutants from the air and provide fresh oxygen for you to breathe. Flowers add color and fragrance to your environment, making your living space more relaxing and enjoyable. Ficus and spider plants are particularly good air filters. Lilies and roses have fragrant aromas that can permeate an entire apartment.

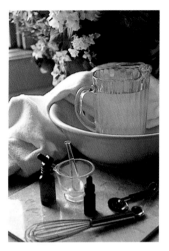

To create these home spa recipes, you will need the following items:

knives

forks

mixing spoons

measuring cups and spoons

eyedropper

small whisk

mixing bowls

blender or food processor

small jars with secure lids

pots with lids

strainer

cotton balls

cotton towels

shower cap

disposable plastic gloves

assorted storage containers

The tools you will need are all common utensils that you probably already have or can easily obtain. Clean and dry each item before and after use. Use plastic, ceramic, enamel, or glass utensils whenever possible, as metals have a tendency to react with certain ingredients.

EQUIPMENT & INGREDIENTS

All ingredients used in the following recipes should be at room temperature, unless otherwise noted. Be sure to use only fresh fruits, vegetables, juices, and dairy products. If something is old or smells funky, don't use it. If you can't find a particular ingredient at your local drugstore, supermarket, or natural foods store, refer to the source guide on page 82. All the recipes in this book make one generous application, unless otherwise noted. You can double or triple any of the recipes and keep extra portions in clean glass or plastic containers.

Each recipe will tell you whether your leftover treatment requires refrigeration. Do not keep those that do need refrigeration for more than three days.

Essential oils, listed as ingredients for many of the recipes in this book, are concentrated plant extracts, available at natural foods stores and aromatherapy shops. In many of the recipes, specific oils are called for because of their individual properties and effects. But every person responds differently to any given scent, so feel free to substitute your favorite. A list on page 81 describes the therapeutic effects of some essential oils. Please note that these oils should not be taken internally or applied to the skin in pure concentration and that excessive use of certain essential oils —like excessive use of anything—is potentially harmful. All the recipes in this book have been tested and none contain dangerous amounts of any ingredient. If you have questions about certain oils, and especially if you are pregnant or have very sensitive skin, be sure to consult a doctor, herbalist, or aromatherapist before use.

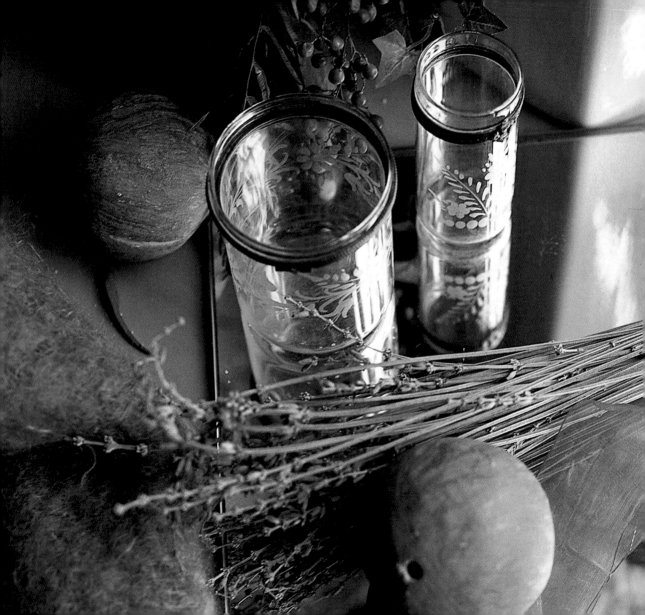

BEFORE YOU BEGIN

There are three things you should know before you begin pampering yourself:

• Some people have more sensitive skin than others. Before treating yourself with any of the mixtures in this book, first apply a small amount of the finished product to the inside of your arm. Wait 24 hours to make sure no rash or other allergic reaction develops.

• Always focus on the part of your body you are attending to. While applying your facial mask, don't think about tomorrow's lunch meeting; think about your skin and your pores. Relax and take the events in your life one at a time.

• Don't rush. If you know you only have ten minutes, treat yourself to a ten-minute foot rub. Don't try to fit in a two-hour facial—you'll only be frustrated. Remember, this should not be work, but relaxation.

Enjoy yourself. When you take the time for your physical well-being, you nourish yourself mentally and emotionally too.

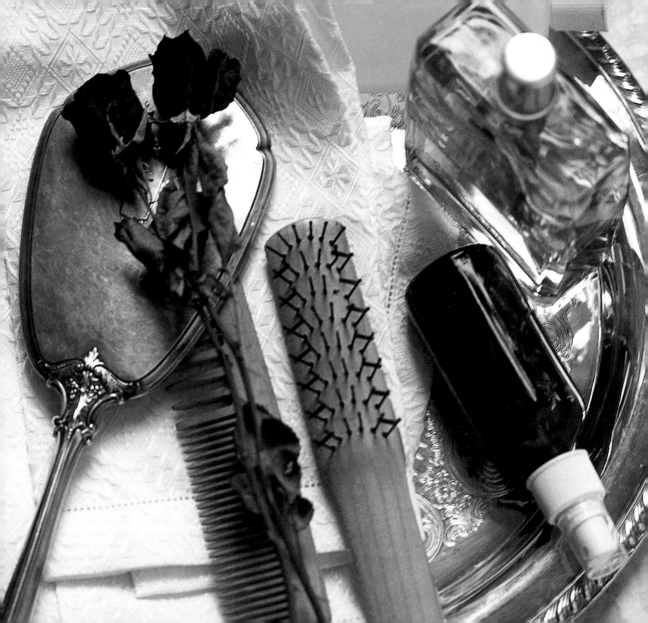

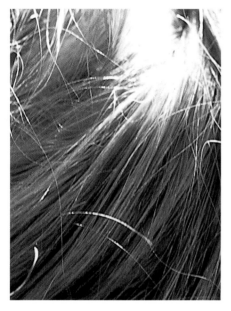

HAIR

While proper cleaning and conditioning is your best protection from the environmental and emotional stresses that attack your hair, manufactured hair products that contain harsh, stripping chemicals can do more harm than good. Be sure your hair is protected by using natural products like those in the following recipes.

rose oil SHAMPOO

Jojoba oil, which is actually a liquid wax, has properties similar to those of our body's natural oils and is ideal as a natural moisture restorer for hair and body. Store in a glass or plastic container in a cool, dry place. Shake gently before using, as mixture will separate as it sits.

½ cup (120 ml) distilled water

½ cup (120 ml) liquid soap or unscented shampoo

1 teaspoon jojoba oil

⅛ teaspoon rose oil

½ teaspoon salt

In a bowl, gently whisk together water and soap or shampoo. Add oils and salt and combine well. Use as you would your regular shampoo.

lemon-herb SHAMPOO

In this shampoo, jojoba oil restores moisture to the hair as lemon oil invigorates and herbs soothe. Store in a glass or plastic container in a cool, dry place. Shake gently before using, as mixture will separate as it sits.

½ cup (120 ml) distilled water

2 tablespoons dried rosemary (dark hair) or chamomile (light hair)

½ cup (120 ml) liquid soap or unscented shampoo

1 teaspoon jojoba oil

¼ teaspoon lemon oil

1 tablespoon salt

In covered pot, heat water and herbs to boiling. Remove from heat and let cool. Strain out herbs and discard, then gently whisk soap or shampoo into herb water. Stir in oils and salt. Use as you would your regular shampoo.

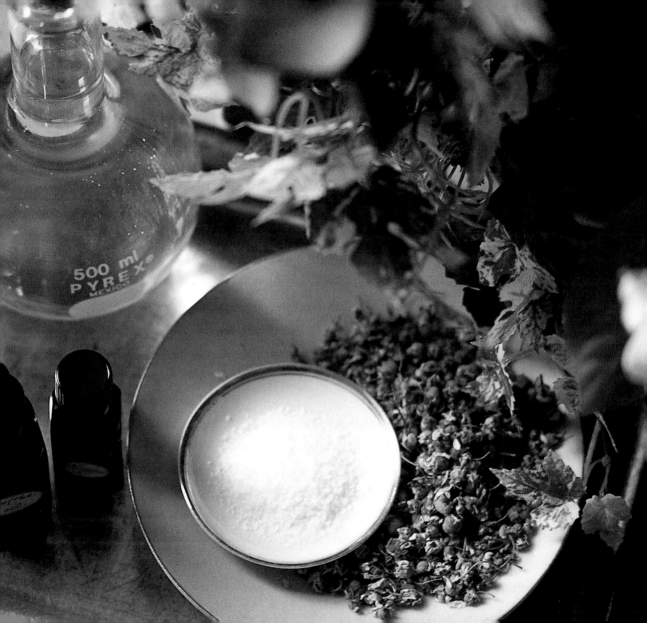

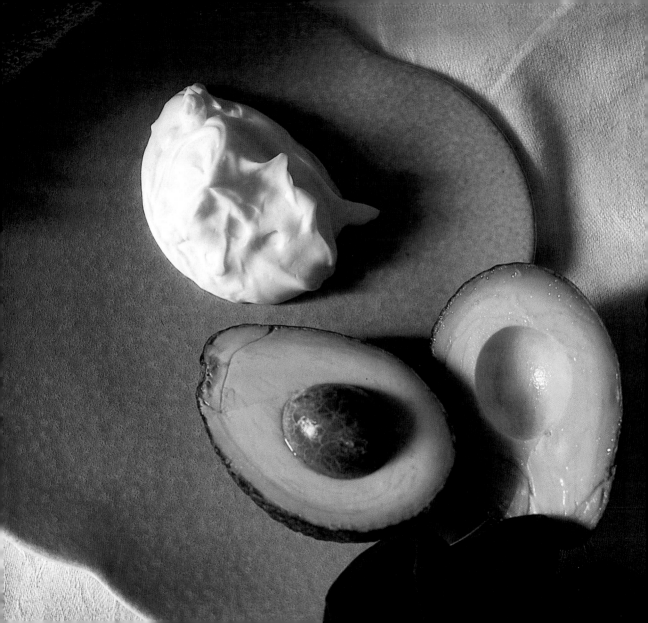

heavy-duty CONDITIONER

The moisturizing properties of the avocado and the conditioning elements of mayonnaise (oil, vinegar, and egg) make this combination an ideal conditioner for dry, brittle hair. Store in a glass or plastic container in the refrigerator.

¼ cup (55 g) mayonnaise

¼ avocado, peeled and mashed

In blender or food processor, combine mayonnaise and avocado until smooth. Massage mixture into hair and scalp. Cover hair with shower cap and leave on 20 minutes. Wash out with gentle shampoo.

deep CONDITIONER

In this all-purpose conditioner, the olive oil conditions and moisturizes your hair while the egg softens it. Store in a glass or plastic container in the refrigerator. Shake before using, as mixture will separate as it sits.

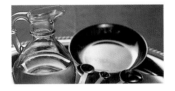

1 teaspoon olive oil

3–4 drops of your favorite essential oil

1 egg, beaten

In a bowl, mix ingredients with whisk or fork. Pour over head and massage into hair and scalp. Cover hair with shower cap and leave on 20 minutes. Wash out with gentle shampoo.

pre-shampoo lemon RINSE

This is the perfect rinse for removing a buildup of styling products before shampooing. Lemon and vodka are natural cleansers. Store in a glass or plastic container in a cool, dry place. Shake before using, as mixture will separate as it sits.

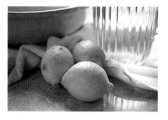

1 cup (230 ml) distilled water
¼ cup (60 ml) vodka
juice of 1 lemon

In a bowl or lidded jar, combine ingredients and stir or shake to mix. Pour rinse through hair before shampooing and conditioning.

herbal final RINSE

This gentle rinse removes buildup as well as any shampoo or conditioner left in hair and leaves hair soft and sweet-smelling. Store in a glass or plastic container in a cool, dry place.

2 cups (460 ml) distilled water
2 tablespoons dried rosemary (dark hair) or chamomile (light hair)

In covered pot, heat water and herbs just to boiling. Remove from heat and let cool. Strain out herbs and discard. Pour rinse through hair after shampooing and conditioning. Pat dry with towel and style as usual.

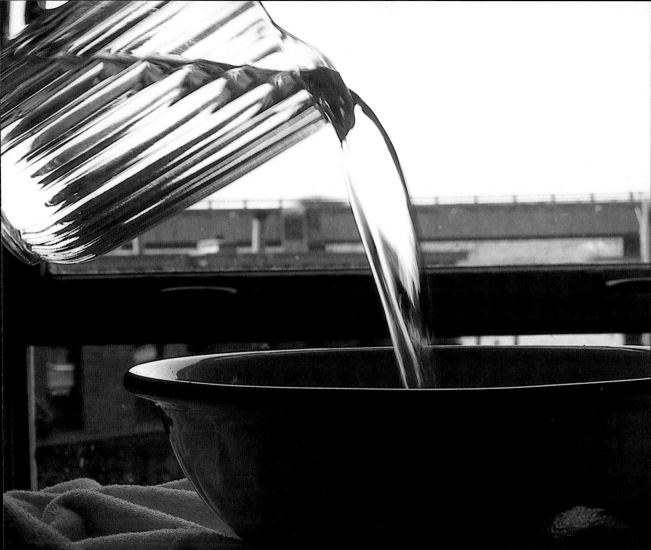

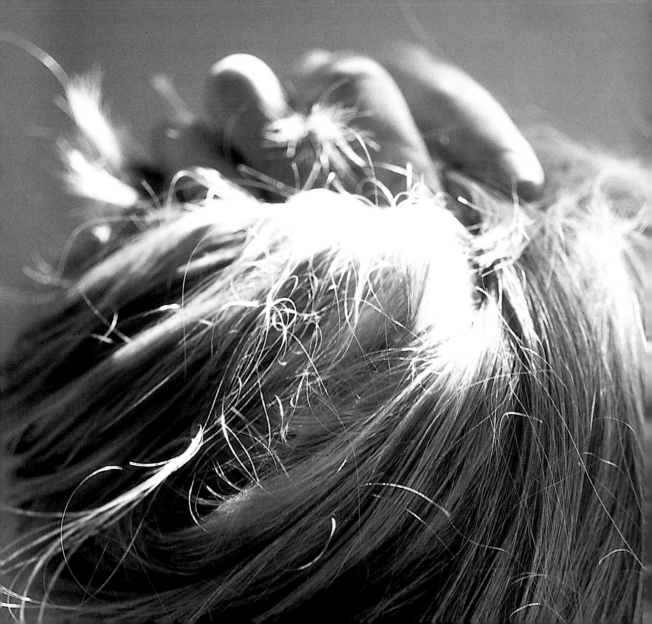

This is a great massage for hair that is styled with gel or spray. Witch hazel gently removes buildup from hair while essential oil protects hair from the sun, wind, and other elements. Store in a glass or plastic container in a cool, dry place. Shake before using, as mixture will separate as it sits.

  I tablespoon witch hazel

  3–4 drops of your favorite essential oil

In small lidded jar, combine witch hazel and oil and shake well. Pour into hands and massage into clean hair and scalp for 3–5 minutes. Style hair as usual.

This is the perfect massage for thin or fine hair. Olive oil softens and conditions while beer adds body and volume. Store in a glass or plastic container in a cool, dry place. Shake before using, as mixture will separate as it sits.

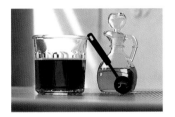

  I cup (230 ml) dark beer

  I teaspoon olive oil

In a bowl, mix beer and oil with whisk or fork. Pour mixture through clean hair and massage into hair and scalp for 3–5 minutes. Rinse hair and style as usual.

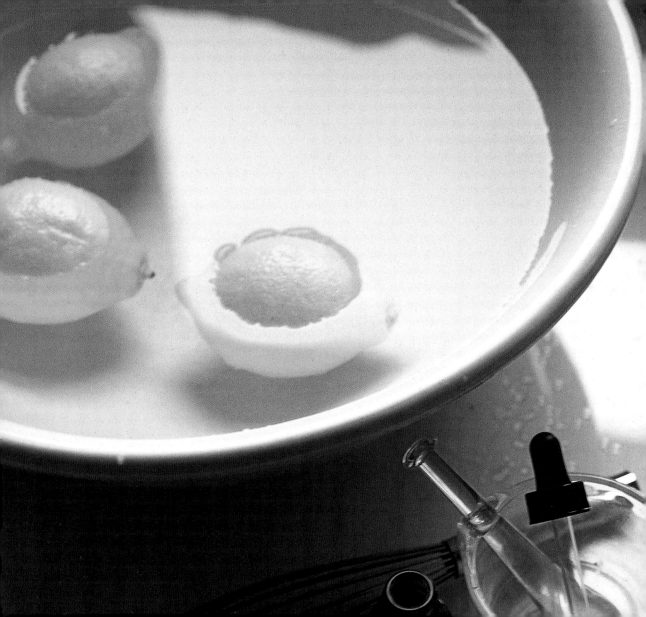

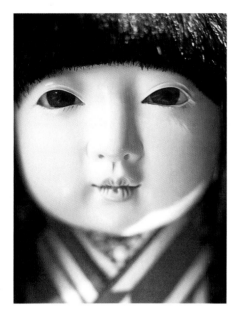

FACE

Your facial skin takes the brunt of environmental battering—sun, wind, and pollution. It suffers further exposure and damage when harsh soaps strip away the natural oils that should protect your skin from the elements. Use the recipes in this section to keep it healthy and well protected. Remember to cleanse your face thoroughly before using any of these masks, and never apply a mask to the area immediately around your eyes.

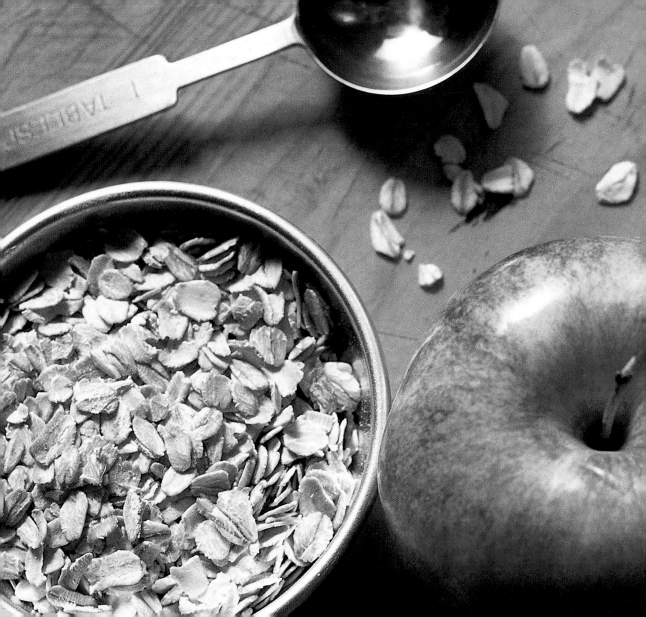

apple-oatmeal SCRUB

Apples are the perfect beauty fruit for all skin types. The apple's juice tightens pores, while its pectin soothes the skin. The exfoliating action of oatmeal and cornmeal in this scrub removes dead skin and improves blood circulation, revealing newer, livelier skin. Store in a glass or plastic container in the refrigerator.

2 tablespoons rolled oats

1 ½ teaspoons cornmeal

1 tablespoon honey

½ medium apple, peeled, cored, and cut into chunks

In a bowl, mix oats, cornmeal, and honey into a paste using a fork. In blender or food processor, combine paste and apple and pulse until smooth. Apply mixture generously to face and gently scrub in circular motion. Rinse off with warm water and pat dry.

strawberry-almond SCRUB

This is the perfect natural scrub for normal to dry skin. Strawberries are an astringent, baking soda a cleanser, almonds an exfoliant, and the combination of yogurt and egg is a moisturizer and skin softener. Store in a glass or plastic container in the refrigerator.

5 strawberries, hulled

1 ½ teaspoons baking soda

1 egg

1 tablespoon vanilla yogurt

¼ cup (40 g) whole almonds with skins

In blender or food processor, combine strawberries, baking soda, egg, and yogurt and blend until smooth. Add almonds and blend until smooth. Apply mixture to face and gently scrub in circular motion. Rinse off with warm water and pat dry.

witch hazel TONER

Perfect for normal to dry skin, this gentle toner leaves face clean and refreshed but not tight or dry. Store in a glass or plastic container in a cool, dry place. Shake before using, as mixture will separate as it sits.

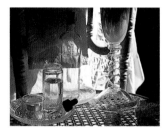

1 teaspoon witch hazel
2–3 drops of your favorite
   essential oil

In small lidded jar, combine witch hazel and oil and shake until oil is dissolved. Soak cotton ball with mixture and gently wipe over face and neck.

cucumber-tomato TONER

This toner is especially good for oily skin. The vegetables and vodka are gentle astringents that remove excess oil and dirt missed in cleansing. Store in a glass or plastic container in the refrigerator.

½ cucumber, cut into chunks
   (do not peel or seed)
½ tomato, cut into chunks
¼ cup (60 ml) vodka

In blender or food processor, combine ingredients and blend until smooth. Dab mixture onto face and neck with fingertips. Toner will be watery, so don't worry if it doesn't seem to adhere to your face. Leave on 3–5 minutes. Rinse off with warm water and pat dry.

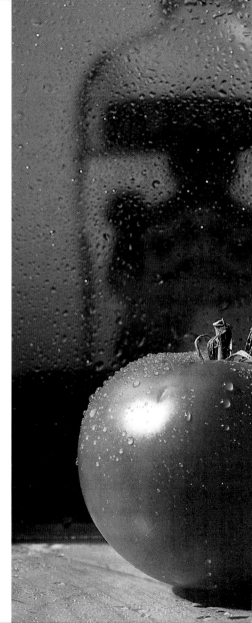

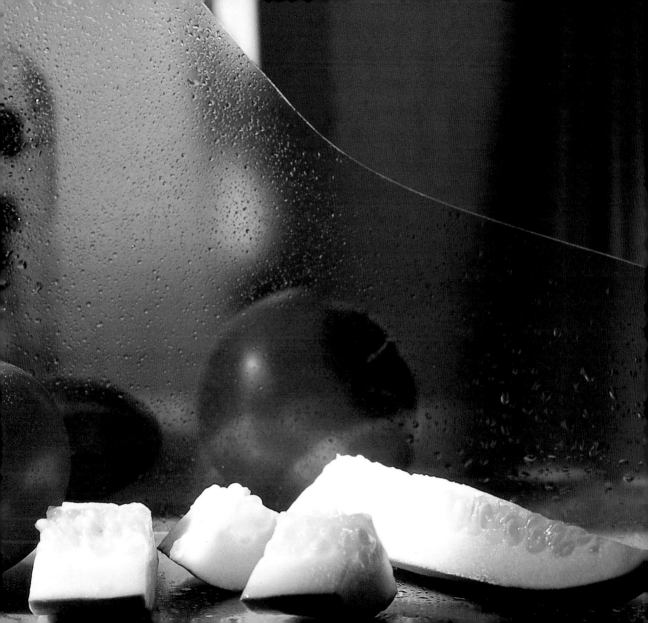

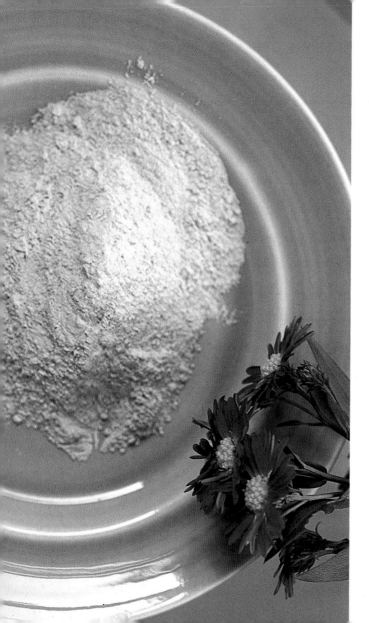

moisturizing MASK

This mask is especially good for dry skin. Avocado, sesame oil, and lactic acid from the yogurt are natural moisturizers. Store in a glass or plastic container in the refrigerator.

1 tablespoon sesame oil
½ soft ripe avocado, peeled
1 tablespoon plain yogurt

In blender or food processor, combine ingredients and blend until smooth. Using circular motion and being careful not to get too close to eyes, massage mask evenly onto face, then leave on 3–5 minutes. Rinse off with warm water and pat dry.

Perfect for oily skin, this mask contains egg white to tone, papaya to exfoliate, and honey to help your skin retain moisture and to prevent it from drying. Although papaya is a very effective beauty aid, it does have a slightly unpleasant smell. Store in a glass or plastic container in the refrigerator.

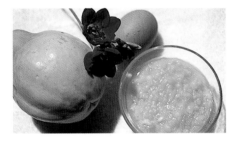

½ ripe papaya, skinned and seeded

1 egg white, beaten

1 teaspoon honey

In a bowl, mash papaya, then stir in egg white. Being careful not to get too close to eyes, apply mask evenly to face and leave on 20 minutes. Rinse off with warm water and pat dry.

The clay in this mask absorbs excess oils and removes dead skin cells while the yogurt and honey moisturize and protect. Store in a glass or plastic container in the refrigerator.

2 teaspoons yogurt

½ teaspoon honey

½ teaspoon cosmetic clay (available at health and natural foods stores)

Combine ingredients and mix thoroughly. Being careful not to get too close to eyes, apply mask evenly to face and leave on 15 minutes. Rinse off with warm water and pat dry.

Steaming opens pores to release impurities missed during regular cleansing. Herbs in the steam soothe the skin and relax the body.

For a mini facial, follow this cleansing steam with your favorite toner from page 30 and your favorite moisturizer from page 37.

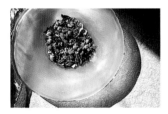

2 quarts (1 liter) distilled water

½ cup (24 g) of your favorite dried herbs (chamomile, sage, peppermint, etc.; can be combined in any proportion)

In covered pot, heat water and herbs to boiling. Remove pot from burner and lid from pot. You may need to let preparation cool a bit. When steam is still hot but not scalding, carefully lean face over pot, draping a towel over your head and the pot. Relax and breathe deeply for at least 5 minutes. Discard preparation when finished.

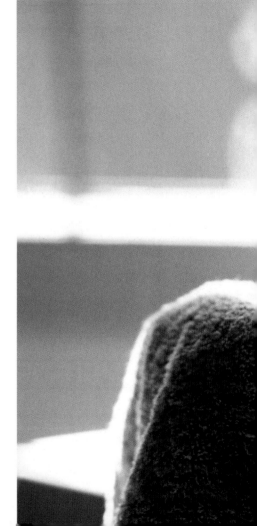

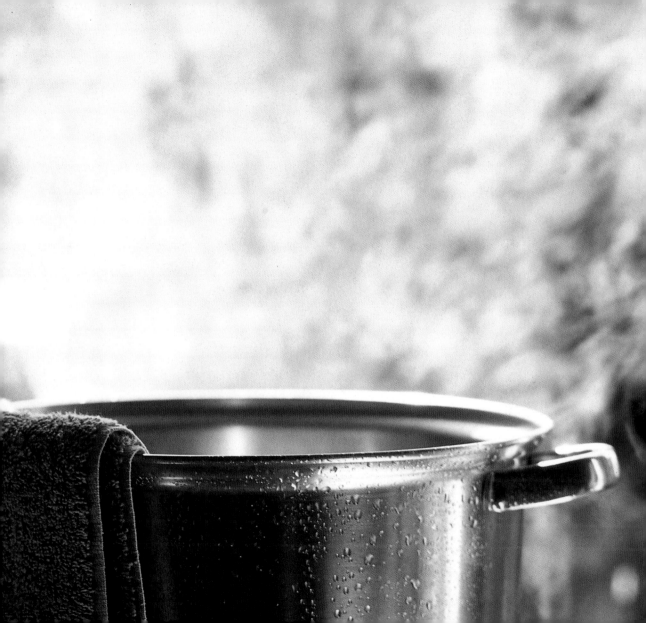

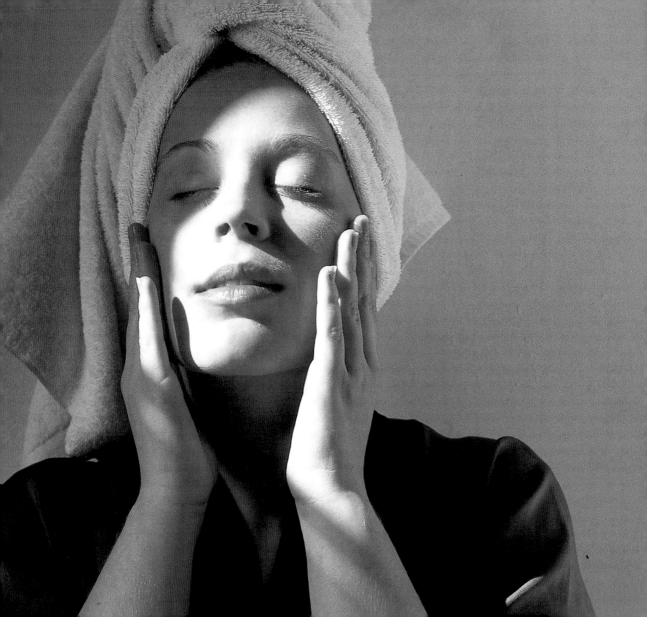

dry skin MOISTURIZER

This is the perfect moisturizer for the winter months. Jojoba oil seals moisture into skin, hydrating and protecting it from harsh external elements. Store in a glass or plastic container in a cool, dry place. Recipe yields several applications.

  2 tablespoons jojoba oil

  7–10 drops of your favorite essential oil

In small lidded jar, combine oils and shake until thoroughly mixed. Apply a few drops to fingertips and massage evenly into face and neck using circular motion.

oily skin light MOISTURIZER

Aloe vera gel is a light, grease-less moisturizer that is perfect for oily skin. Essential oils protect and moisturize. Store in a glass or plastic container in a cool, dry place. Recipe yields several applications.

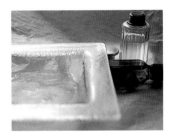

  2 tablespoons aloe vera gel

  7–10 drops of your favorite
    essential oil

In a bowl, combine gel and oil with whisk or fork until well blended. Apply mixture evenly to face and neck using circular motion.

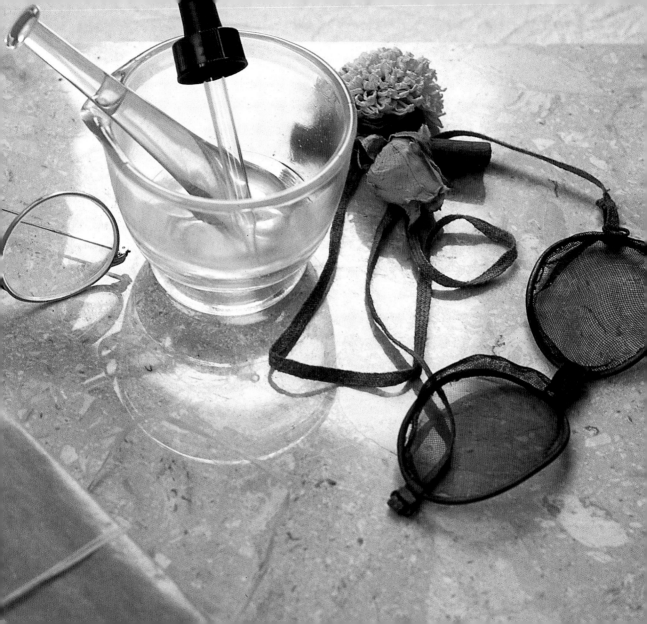

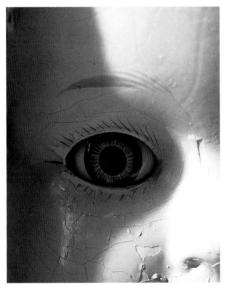

EYES

The skin around your eyes is extremely sensitive, so when your eyes are tired, your whole face looks tired. Taking care of the skin around your eyes can greatly improve your appearance. Because eyes are so sensitive, use toner and moisturizer only around—never on—your eyes.

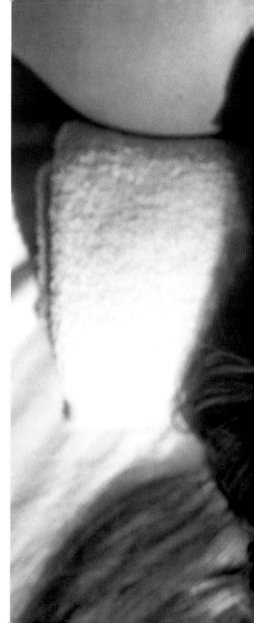

puffiness REDUCER

Turn on your favorite music before you lean back and place the soaked cotton balls over your eyes. This treatment affords you the perfect opportunity to truly listen.

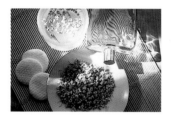

This toner reduces the puffiness of tired eyes. Rose water tones skin and tightens pores while chamomile reduces inflammation. Store in a glass or plastic container in a cool, dry place.

1 bag chamomile tea
1 cup (230 ml) boiling water
½ cup (120 ml) rose water

Steep tea bag in boiling water for 5 minutes. Remove bag and allow tea to cool. Add rose water to tea. Soak two cotton balls in preparation and place over eyelids. Leave on for 5 minutes.

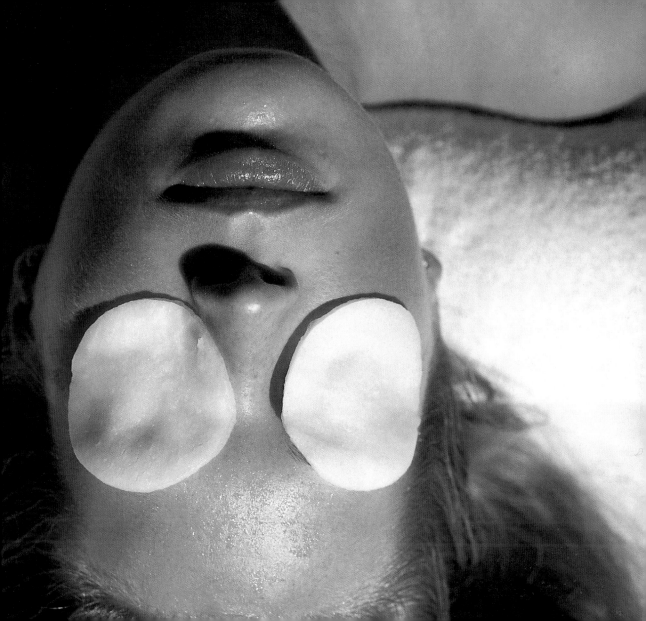

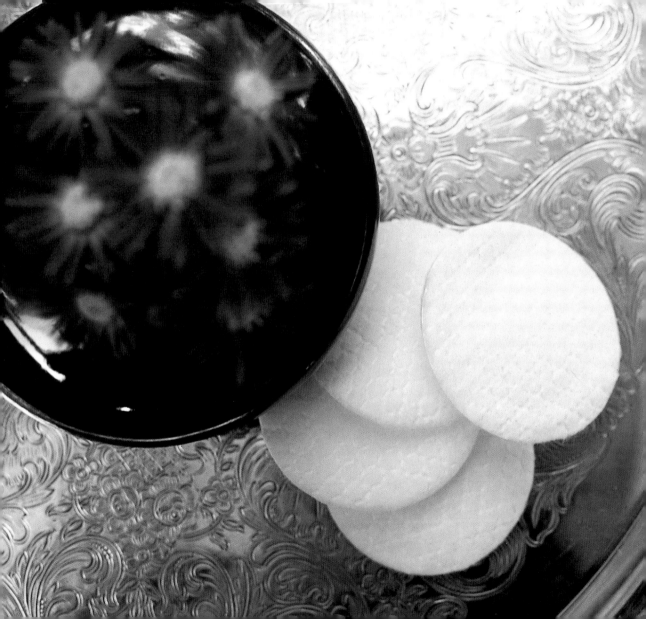

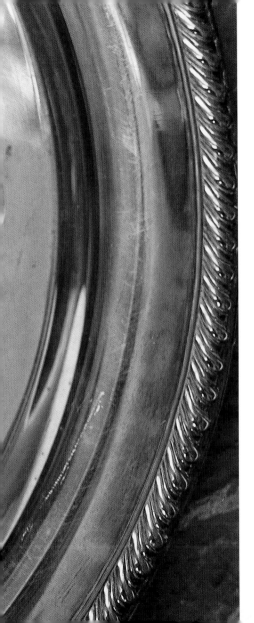

cucumber TONER

The refreshing, gently astrin-gent qualities of cucumber make this a perfect toner for the delicate skin around the eyes. Store in a glass or plastic container in the refrigerator.

½ cucumber, cut into 1-inch (2.5 cm) chunks (do not peel or seed)

3 tablespoons witch hazel

Puree cucumber in blender or food processor until liquefied. Strain through fine mesh, reserving cucumber juice and disposing of pulp and seeds. Mix witch hazel with cucumber juice. Soak cotton ball with mixture and gently wipe around the eye area.

Use this toner on your whole face for a quick, refreshing pick-me-up any time of the day.

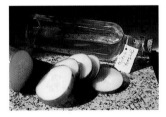

special eye MOISTURIZER

Aloe vera is a light moisturizer that is easily absorbed into the delicate eye area. The anti-inflammatory quality of sesame oil helps reduce puffiness. Store in a glass or plastic container in a cool, dry place. Shake before using, as mixture will separate as it sits. Recipe yields approximately one ounce (28 g) of moisturizer.

Packaged in an elegant glass jar, this luxurious moisturizer makes the perfect gift.

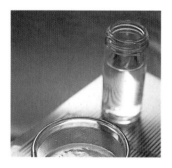

2 tablespoons aloe vera gel
1 tablespoon sesame oil

In a bowl, combine gel and oil with whisk or fork until well blended. Apply mixture evenly in delicate circular motion around eye area.

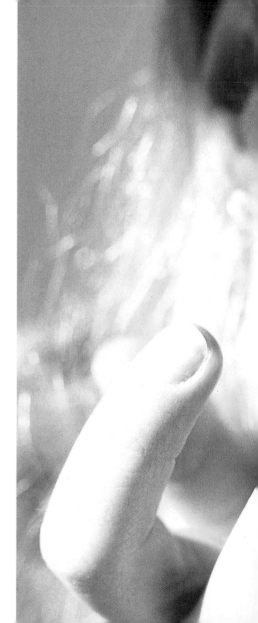

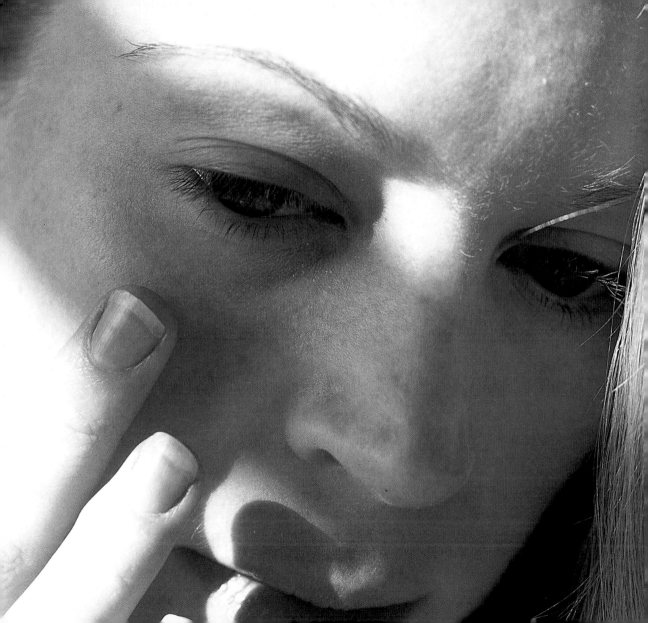

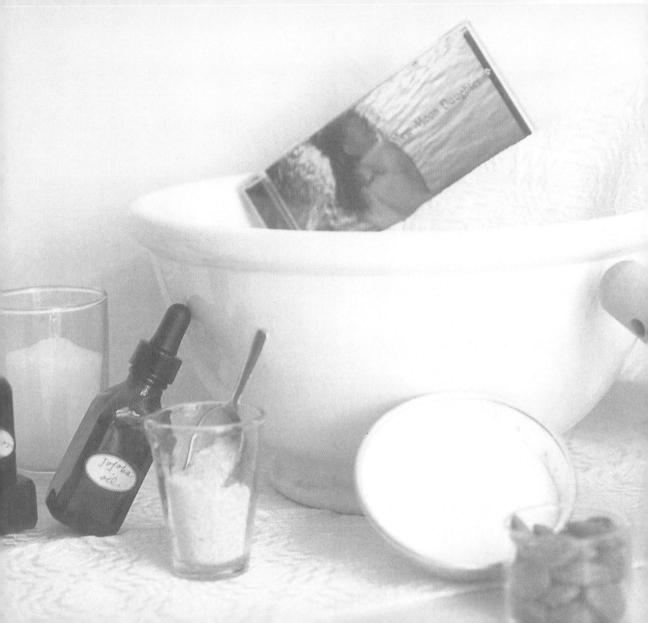

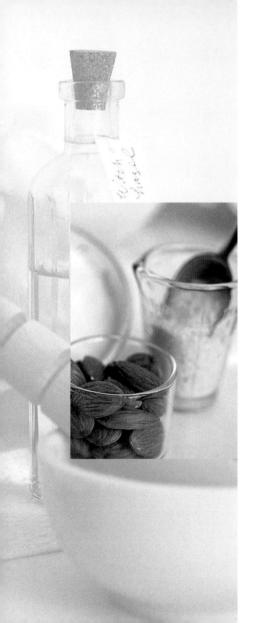

When you have the time to thoroughly enjoy it, treat yourself to a complete facial. The whole process should take approximately two and a half hours, but the longer you stretch it out, the more luxurious it will feel. Make this time as relaxing as possible. Before you begin, light your favorite scented candle and turn on some music you haven't listened to in a while. During the twenty minutes you're sitting with your facial mask on, watch a half-hour television show you've prerecorded or pick up a magazine article you've been meaning to read.

1. Cleanse and exfoliate with Apple-Oatmeal Scrub or Strawberry-Almond Scrub (page 29).

2. To remove any remaining dirt and oil and prepare skin to receive full benefit of facial, tone with Witch Hazel Toner or Cucumber-Tomato Toner (page 30).

3. Moisturize and nourish skin with Moisturizing Mask, Stimulating Mask, or Clay Mask (pages 32–33).

4. Open and cleanse pores and hydrate skin with Herbal Steam (page 34).

5. Moisturize and protect skin with Dry Skin Moisturizer or Oily Skin Light Moisturizer (page 37).

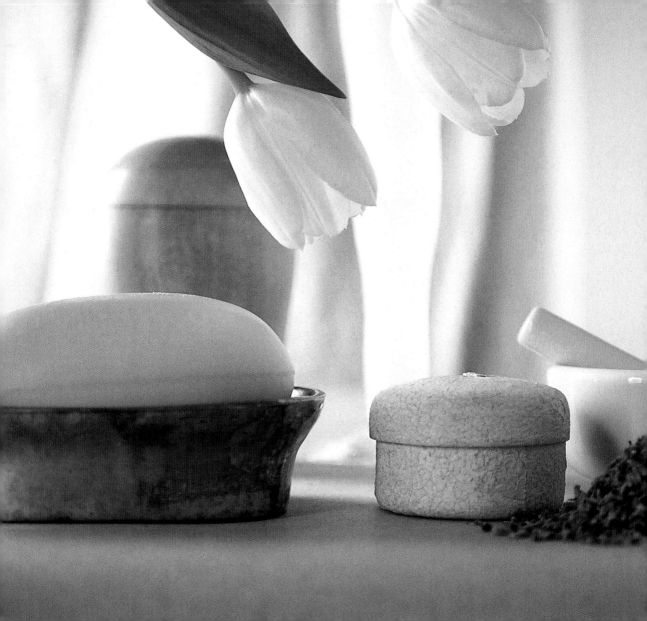

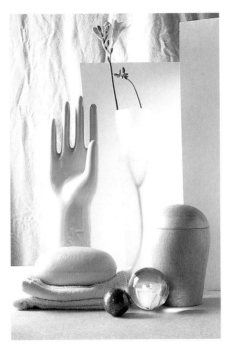

HANDS & NAILS

Some say that your hands tell the story of your life—washing dishes, gardening, fixing your car. Don't let dry, damaged hands and nails reveal your tale! Rehydrate and repair with the following treatments.

buttermilk SOAK

Gentle on hands, buttermilk is a mild exfoliant and an excellent skin conditioner. The lactic acid in buttermilk is said to stimulate nail cell growth. Store in a glass or plastic container in the refrigerator. Shake before using, as mixture will separate as it sits.

½ cup (120 ml) buttermilk

½ cup (120 ml) warm distilled water

1 teaspoon almond oil

In a bowl, combine ingredients with whisk or fork. Soak hands in mixture for 15 minutes. Rinse and pat dry with towel.

super cuticle SOFTENER

Massaging the cuticle area and keeping it moisturized and hydrated maintains healthy nails and encourages new nail growth. Store in a glass or plastic container in a cool, dry place.

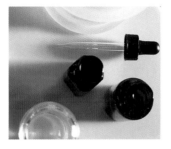

1 teaspoon olive oil

1 teaspoon vitamin E oil

Combine ingredients and massage into nails and cuticles.

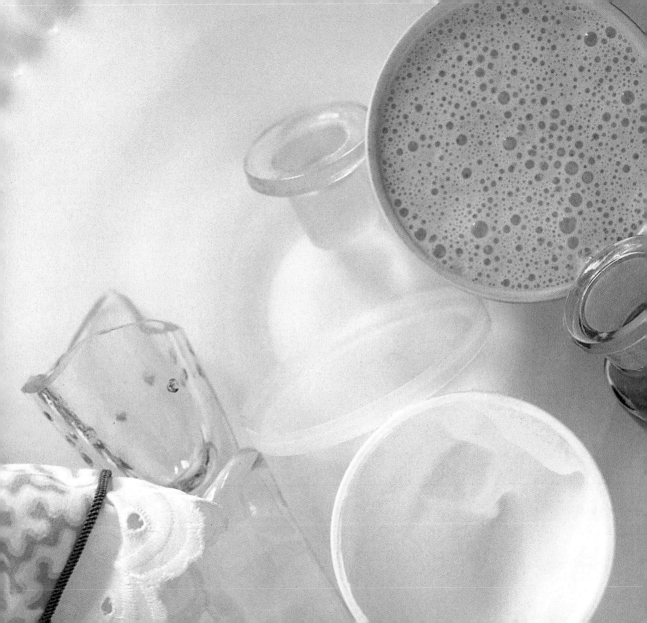

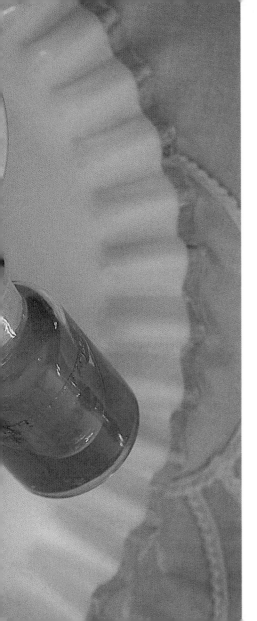

MASK

A healing mask for overworked hands, this recipe is not only effective but smells great! Apricots contain vitamin A, which helps heal damaged cells in the top layer of skin. Yogurt and honey soften and moisturize. Store in a glass or plastic container in the refrigerator.

Ask a friend to join you in the hand mask treatment. It's a perfect opportunity for you to spend relaxing, quality time together.

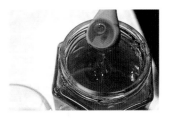

¼ cup (50 g) dried apricots
¼ cup (60 ml) plain yogurt
I tablespoon honey

In blender or food processor, combine ingredients and blend until smooth. Spread mask onto hands and nails and leave on 20 minutes. You may want to wear disposable plastic gloves while the mask sits. Rinse with warm water and pat dry.

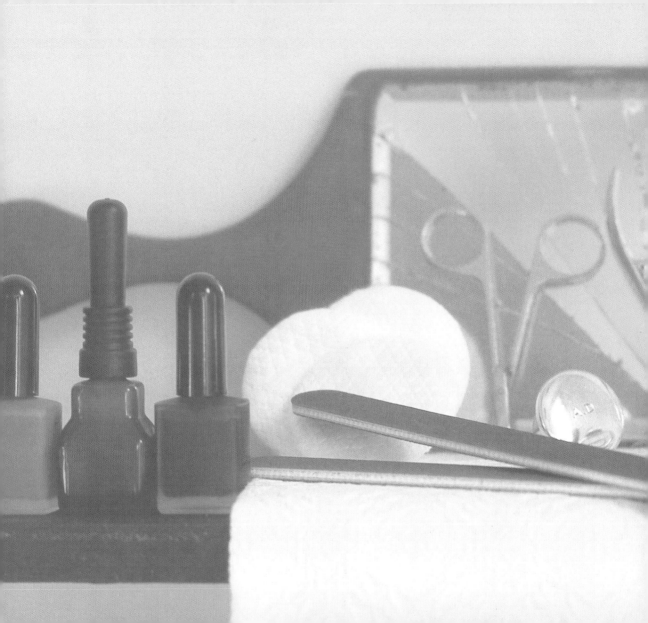

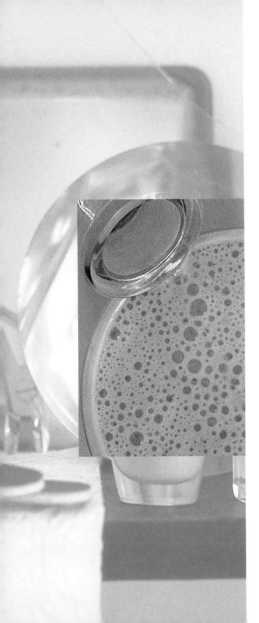

A manicure is especially fun to do with a friend. During the Buttermilk Soak and the Apricot Hand Mask, you'll have plenty of time to catch up on each other's lives, a pleasure we seem to find less and less time for. Make up the recipes in advance so you are ready to begin when your friend arrives. Flowers will make your environment particularly aromatic and inviting. The whole process should take approximately an hour and a half to two hours, but you may want it to never end!

1. Remove any polish from nails.

2. Lightly and evenly file nails with emery board so they are smooth and gently rounded.

3. Soak nails in Buttermilk Soak (page 51).

4. Apply Super Cuticle Softener (page 51) and gently push cuticles back from nails with cotton-covered wooden cuticle stick.

5. Apply Apricot Hand Mask (page 53).

6. Moisturize hands with your favorite hand lotion.

7. Make sure hands and nails are thoroughly dry, then apply base coat followed by two coats of your favorite nail polish. Seal the polish with top coat. Wait 10 minutes between coats.

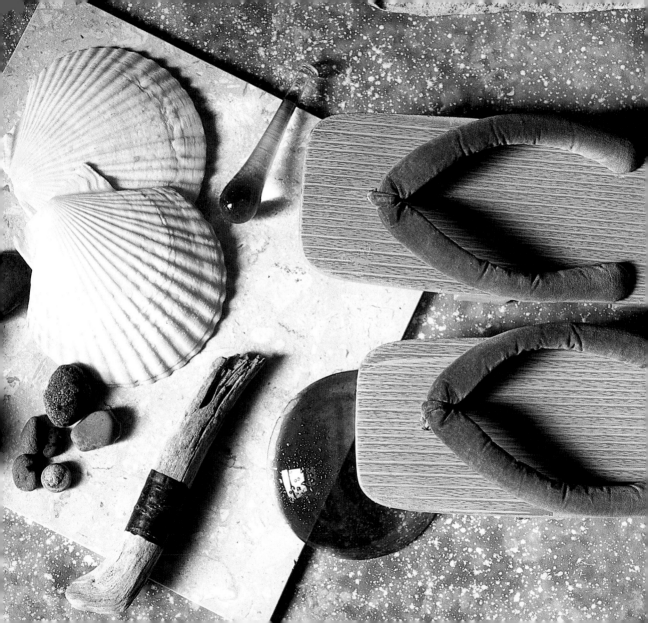

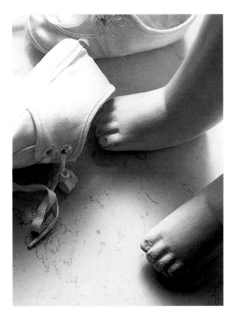

FEET

If there is one part of your body that you neglect in your beauty regimen, it's probably your feet. With the miles they take you and the shoes you squeeze them into, they deserve just as much if not more attention than other parts of your body. Treat your feet right with the following recipes.

Next time you take a trip to the beach, bring home a container of sand for this foot scrub. Each time you use it to soften your feet, you'll be reminded of your time at the beach.

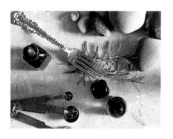

Sand is a very effective exfoliant for the tough skin that develops on feet. Canola oil softens as rosemary oil invigorates. Store in a glass or plastic container in a cool, dry place.

2 tablespoons canola oil
2 tablespoons beach sand
3–5 drops rosemary oil

Combine ingredients and mix into a paste using a fork. Massage scrub onto feet, concentrating especially on problem areas, like heels. Rinse off with warm water and pat dry.

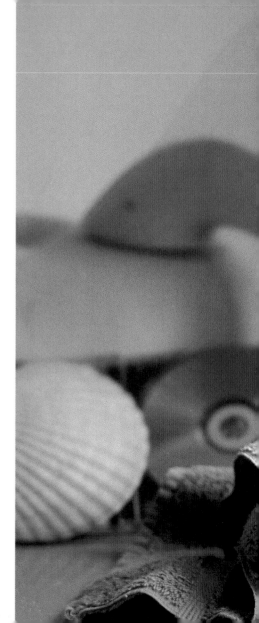

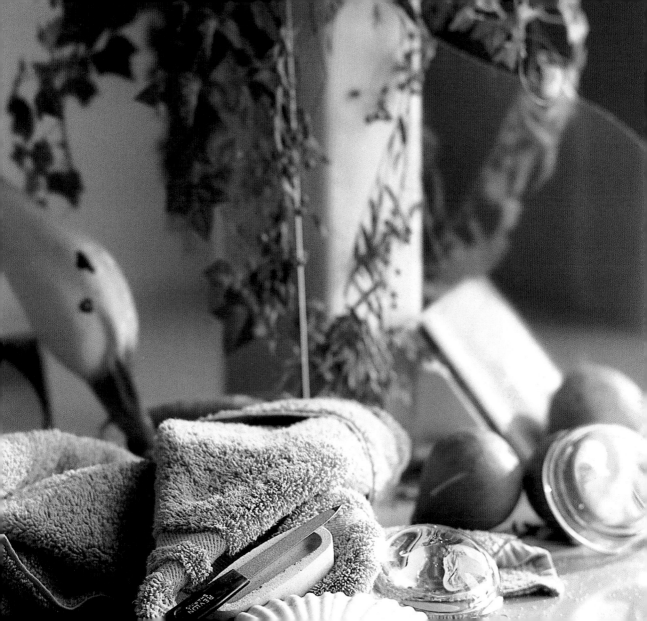

clove oil foot RUB

Clove oil is an astringent with mild anesthetic qualities that soothes tired feet. Sesame oil is an anti-inflammatory. Store in a glass or plastic container in a cool, dry place.

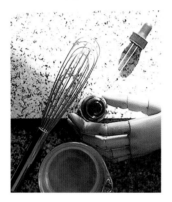

1 teaspoon clove oil

1 teaspoon sesame oil

Combine oils with whisk or fork and massage mixture into feet until absorbed.

peppermint oil foot RUB

This rub is the perfect pick-me-up for tired feet. Peppermint oil stimulates, while aloe vera cools and moisturizes without greasiness. Store in a glass or plastic container in a cool, dry place.

2 tablespoons aloe vera gel

½ tablespoon peppermint oil

Combine ingredients with whisk or fork and massage mixture into feet until absorbed.

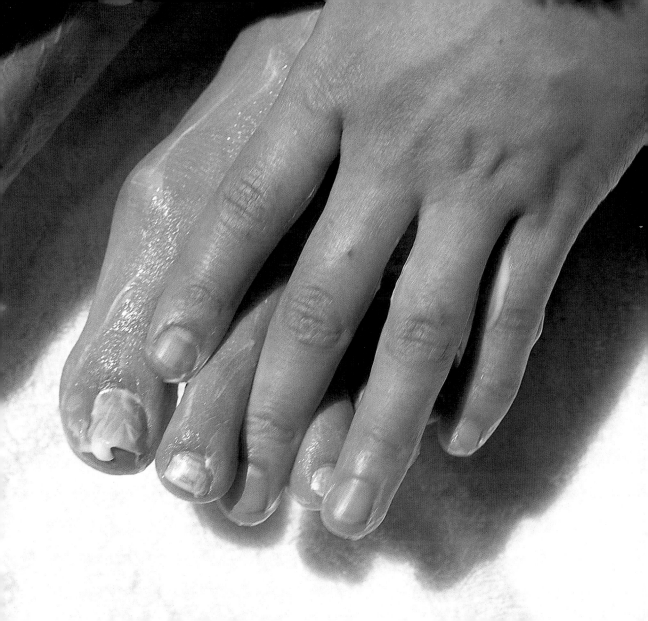

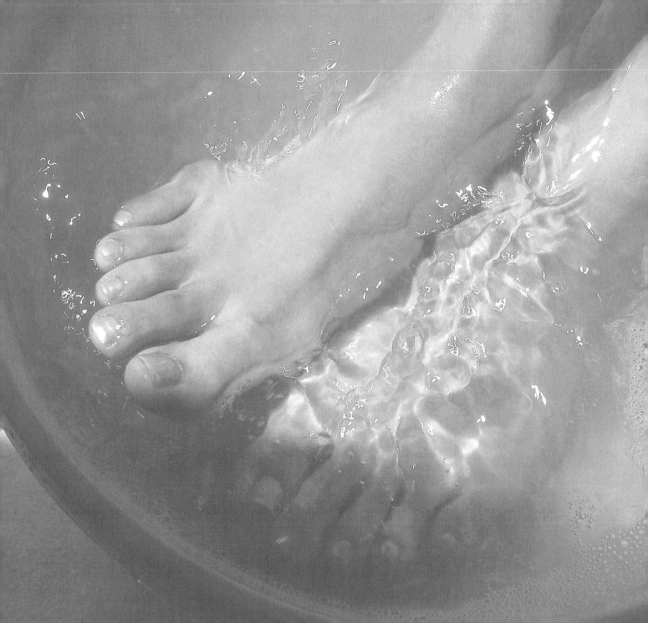

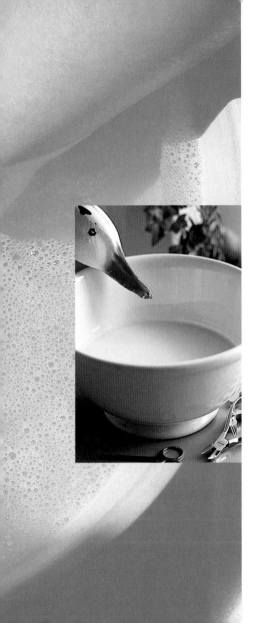

There is something intensely personal about a pedicure. For this reason it is one of the most luxurious gifts you can give yourself, and you should go all out. Put on your silkiest robe, light some incense, and brew yourself a cup of soothing tea. As you soak your feet, sit back and listen to your most romantic album. The whole pedicure should take approximately one hour.

1. Remove any polish from nails.

2. Soak feet for 15 minutes in your favorite bath soak or Buttermilk Soak for hands (page 51). Apply Super Cuticle Softener (page 51) and gently push cuticles back from nails with cotton-covered wooden cuticle stick. Pat dry with towel.

3. Remove dry, dead skin with Beach Sand Foot Scrub (page 58). Rinse off with warm water and pat dry with towel.

4. Clip nails straight across with sharp toenail clippers or scissors.

5. Lightly file nails smooth with emery board.

6. Massage Clove Oil Foot Rub or Peppermint Oil Foot Rub (page 60) into feet. Take your time and massage deeply.

7. Make sure feet and nails are thoroughly dry, then apply base coat followed by two coats of your favorite nail polish. Seal the polish with top coat. Wait 10 minutes between coats.

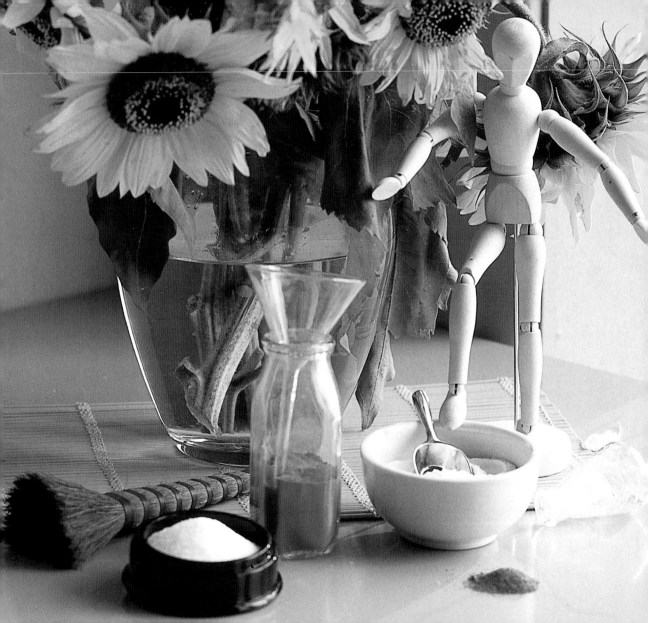

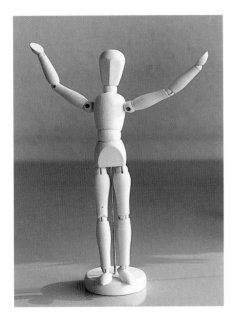

BODY

Too often we think of our bodies in parts, treating only sections while neglecting to treat the whole. Ask a friend or partner to give you a massage with one of the following oils or help you with the body wrap. Your entire being will feel calm and refreshed.

Sesame oil is an anti-inflammatory and thus the perfect massage oil for tired, overworked muscles. Eucalyptus cools and soothes. Store in a glass or plastic container in a cool, dry place.

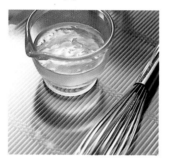

¼ cup (60 ml) sesame oil

½ teaspoon eucalyptus oil

Combine oils with whisk or fork. Use liberally during massage.

The warm, sweet scent of this oil relaxes the mind while the anti-inflammatory qualities of the cinnamon and the sesame oil soothe skin and muscles. Store in a glass or plastic container in a cool, dry place.

¼ cup (60 ml) sesame oil

2 tablespoons almond oil

¼ teaspoon ground cinnamon

¼ teaspoon ground nutmeg

Combine ingredients with whisk or fork, then let stand for at least 3 hours. Strain mixture into jar through paper coffee filter or paper towel to remove ground spices. Use liberally during massage.

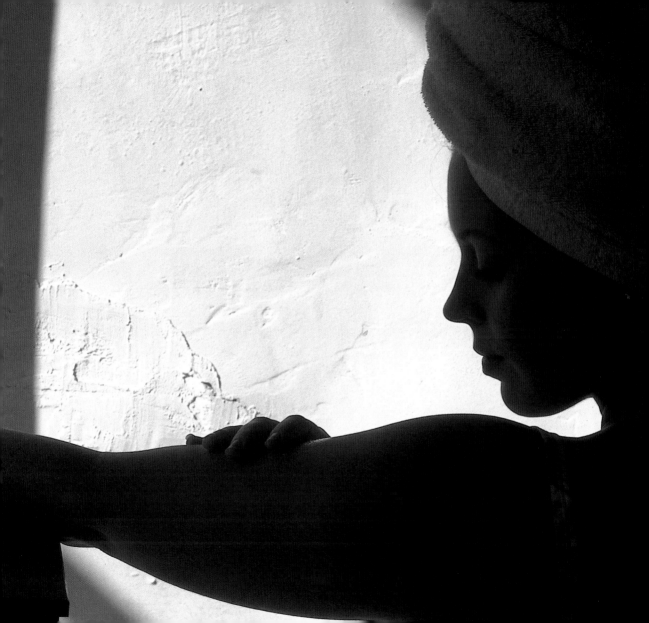

body-buffing salt SCRUB

Salt rubs, popular in spas around the world, exfoliate skin as they stimulate circulation in the body. Store in a glass or plastic container in a cool, dry place.

For a rejuvenating and relaxing full-body treatment, follow this salt scrub with your favorite bath from page 71.

3 cups (725 g) coarse kosher salt

1 cup (230 ml) safflower oil

7–10 drops of your favorite essential oil

Combine ingredients into a paste and rub onto skin all over body except face and neck. Rinse off with warm water and pat dry.

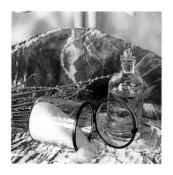

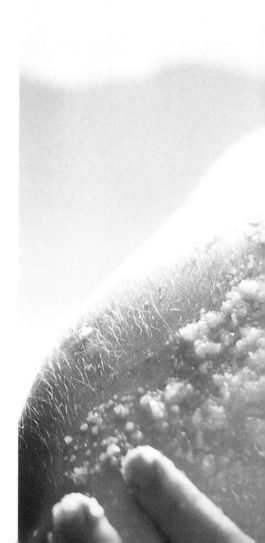

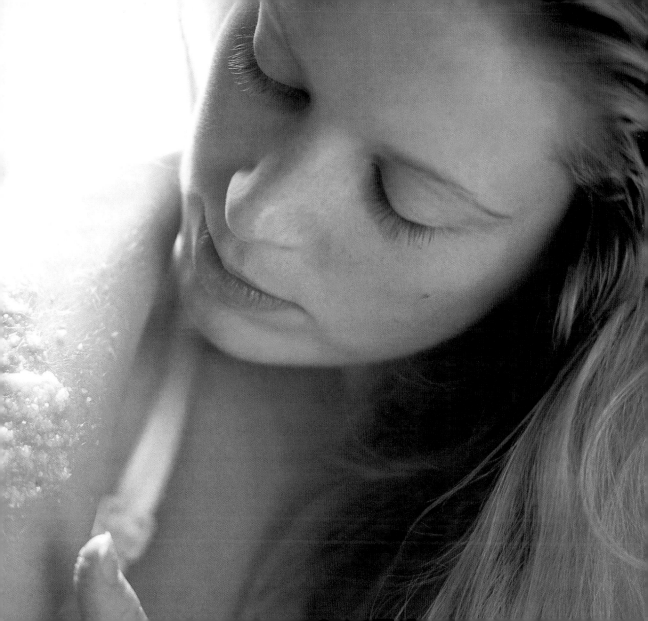

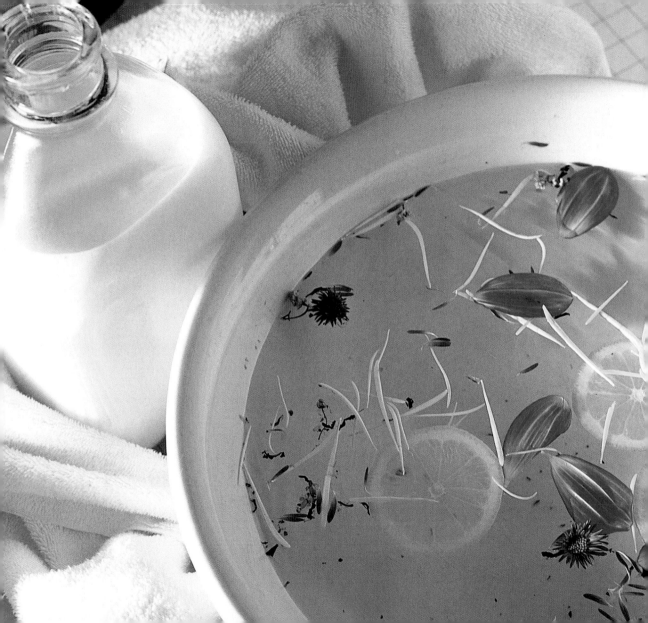

skin-softening milk BATH

Rich milk baths have been used to soften skin since the days of Cleopatra. Honey seals in moisture and protects skin. Store in a glass or plastic container in a cool, dry place.

½ cup (40 g) powdered milk

¼ cup (34 g) cornstarch

¼ cup (60 ml) honey

5–7 drops rose oil

2–3 tablespoons distilled water

In blender or food processor, combine powdered milk, cornstarch, honey, and rose oil. Add distilled water slowly until mixture becomes a smooth paste. Add to running bathwater. Soak for 10–20 minutes.

sore-muscle BATH

Epsom salts have long been used to soothe sore muscles. Jojoba moisturizes, and lavender calms the senses. Store in a glass or plastic container in a cool, dry place.

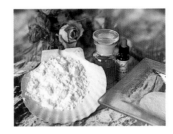

1 cup (250 g) epsom salts

1 teaspoon jojoba oil

5–7 drops lavender oil

Combine ingredients and add to running bathwater. Soak for 10–20 minutes.

seaweed body WRAP

Seaweed firms and moisturizes skin. Enlist the help of a friend, as a body wrap treatment is difficult to perform alone.

1 cup (25 g) dried seaweed or powdered kelp or 2 cups (250 g) fresh seaweed

3 gallons (11 liters) distilled water

1 large beach towel

1 large plastic garbage bag, cut open into large rectangle

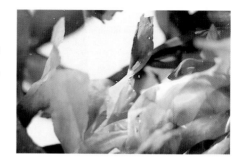

In a large kettle of very hot water, steep seaweed or kelp for 5 minutes. Pour preparation into bathroom sink or bathtub with drain closed. Drop in towel and let it absorb the mixture. Wring out towel and wrap around your body, making sure to enclose as much seaweed as possible. With assistance, wrap the opened plastic bag completely around you and the hot towel. Lie down and relax for 15 minutes. In the bathtub, slowly unwrap yourself and rinse off. Skin-softening Milk Bath (page 71) is a sweet smelling, relaxing way to remove any lingering seaweed scent. Discard leftover preparation.

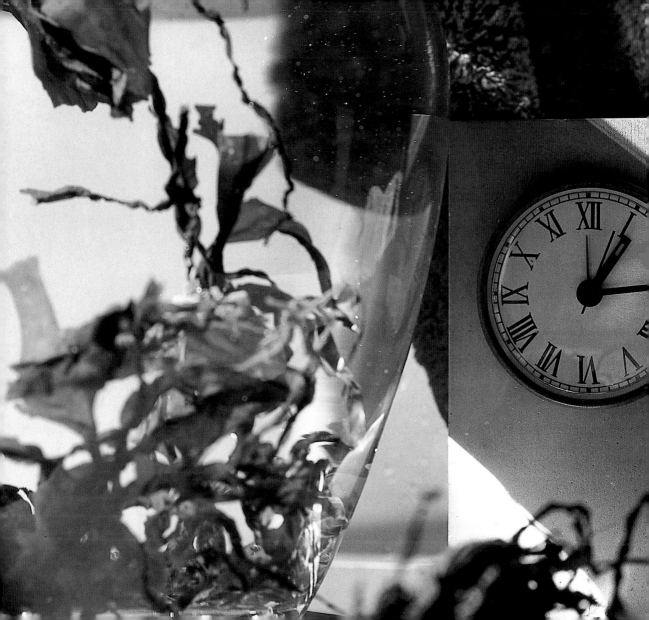

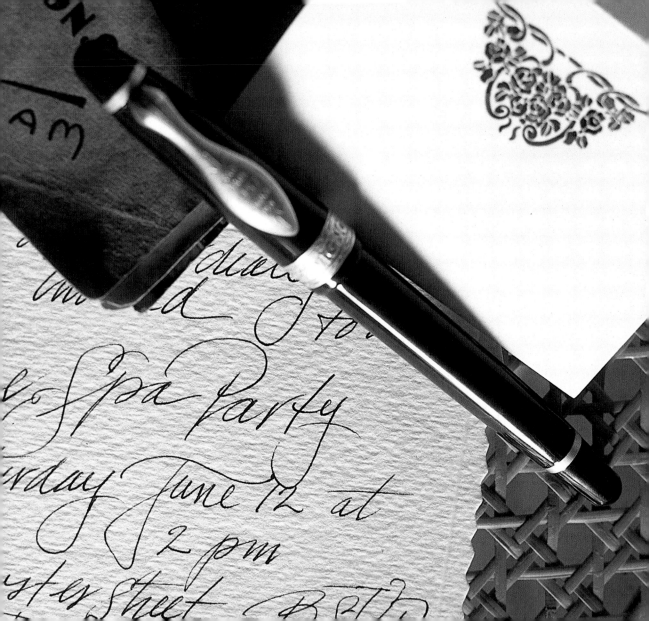

SPA PARTIES

Now that you know just how beneficial the formulas in this book are to your mind and body, you can share them with your friends. Once you've mastered the art of creating the perfect home spa environment and feel comfortable preparing these recipes, try hosting a spa party. Your party can be theme-based, can accompany a holiday or special event, or can replace the traditional bridal or baby shower. Ask each of your guests to bring a spa treatment they've made, or prepare a number of recipes in advance and supply everything yourself. Your party will live on after the event if you prepare a large quantity of an oil or shampoo that will keep without refrigeration, package it in attractive containers, and give one to each guest as a parting gift. Following are a few spa party suggestions.

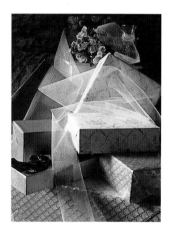

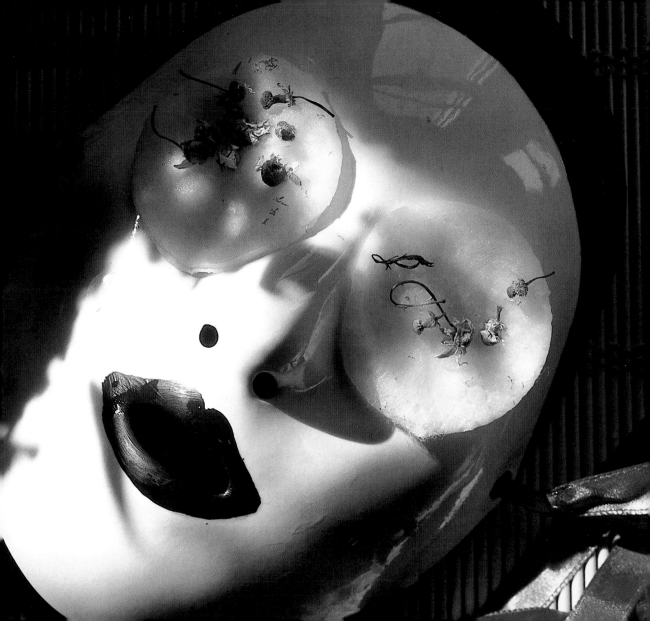

Invite a group of friends to your home and ask each one to bring a bouquet of flowers, a light cotton or silk robe, a pair of thong slippers, and their favorite nail polish. Turn on some light music, and when your guests arrive, relax in your robes with peppermint iced tea. Then start the party with the Ultimate Facial (page 47), followed by the Ultimate Pedicure (page 63). After your spa treatments, lounge surrounded by bouquets of flowers and music with more iced tea, light sandwiches, and fruit salad.

Give the gift of beauty and relaxation to a few of your closest friends. Have them bring thick robes and their favorite slippers to the party. Welcome them into your home with a fire in the fireplace, if you have one, the warm glow of lanterns, and the scent of pine. Start the party by relaxing in your robes with a pot of spicy orange tea and opera or Christmas music. Then begin your spa treatments with Conditioning Scalp Massage (page 25), followed by Rose Oil Shampoo (page 18) and Herbal Final Rinse (page 22). Next, treat winter-battered

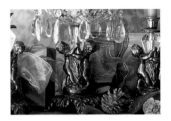

skin with Apple-Oatmeal Scrub (page 29) and Moisturizing Mask (page 32). When you and your friends are relaxed and refreshed, sit back down to more tea and homemade Christmas cookies. Send your guests home with gift bottles of Rose Oil Shampoo.

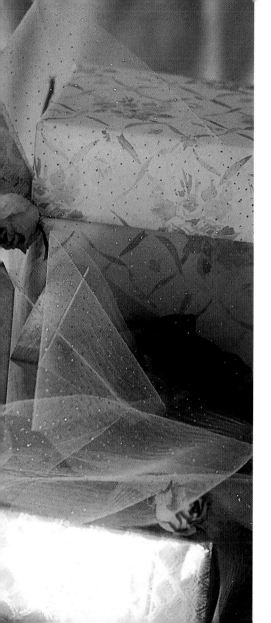

Instead of throwing a typical shower for a friend who is getting married, throw a spa shower. Have your friends make massage oils, scrubs, moisturizers, and shampoos that do not require refrigeration and package them in pretty jars to give as presents. These gifts are much more personal than store-bought items.

Alternatively, plan a full day of spa treatment for your soon-to-be-married friend. Assign specific tasks or recipes to other friends. For example, one can be responsible for all recipes for the Ultimate Manicure (page 55), another can be responsible for the Ultimate Pedicure (page 63), and so on. At the shower, you can all join in treating your friend to the ultimate in relaxation and pampering—a treat far more special than an impersonal day at a professional spa, surrounded by people she doesn't know.

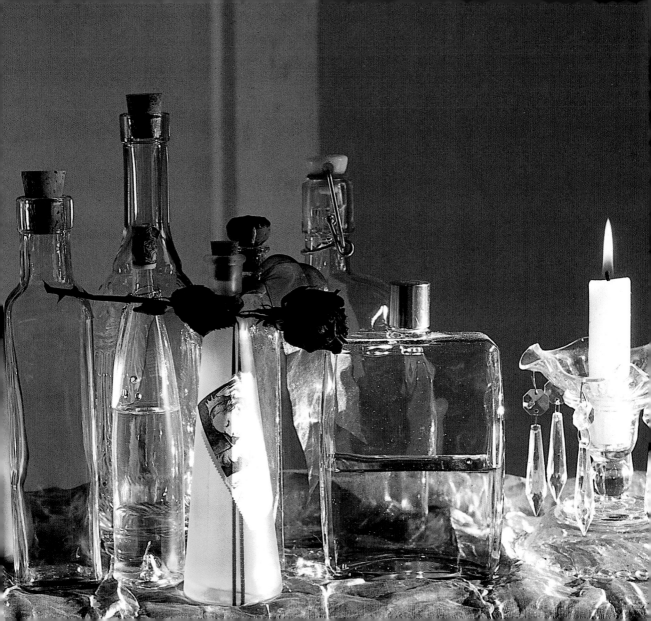

SCENTS

The recent popularity of aromatherapy —the use of essential plant oils to achieve or enhance physical and emotional well-being—has confirmed what most health and beauty experts have known for decades: There is power in natural scents. The aromas of certain plants and herbs can be used to calm, energize, balance, and heal. Adding essential oils to the recipes in this book will increase the calming and beautifying qualities of the treatments. You can also enhance the quality of your environment by applying a few drops of essential oil to potpourri, bathwater, a burning candle, or a light bulb. Following is a list of essential oils and their generally recognized effects. Response to aroma is, of course, individual. Follow your nose!

Bay: invigorates and refreshes

Chamomile: calms and relaxes, soothes physical and emotional distress

Clary sage: relaxes; counters insomnia

Eucalyptus: invigorates and refreshes

Ginger: energizes

Lavender: calms and balances emotions; counters insomnia

Lemon: refreshes, sharpens the senses; uplifts emotionally

Nutmeg: invigorates

Patchouli: arouses sexual desire

Peppermint: invigorates and stimulates

Pine: warms and invigorates

Rose: calms and relaxes; uplifts emotionally

Rosemary: invigorates and stimulates

Thyme: relaxes

Ylang-ylang: soothes, balances, arouses sexual desire

SOURCE GUIDE

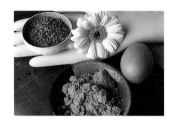

The recipes in this book were chosen not only for their healing and restorative properties, but also for their readily available ingredients. If, for some reason, you cannot find an ingredient at your local drugstore, supermarket, or natural foods store, following is a list of mail-order suppliers around the country who would be happy to send you what you need.

Aroma Vera
5901 Rodeo Road
Los Angeles, CA 90016-4312
800-669-9514
essential oils, unscented shampoos

The Body Shop
45 Horsehill Road
Cedar Knolls, NJ 07927-2014
800-541-2535
fragrance oils, unscented shampoos

General Bottle Supply
P.O. Box 58734
Vernon, CA 90058-0734
jars, containers

Herb Products Company
P.O. Box 898
N. Hollywood, CA 91603-0898
213-877-3104
fragrance oils, botanical products

Kiehl's, Inc.
109 Third Avenue
New York, NY 10003
800-543-4571
fragrance oils, unscented shampoos

Santa Fe Fragrance Consultants
P.O. Box 282
Santa Fe, NM 87504
(please send self-addressed stamped envelope for catalog)
essential oils

Tenzing Momo
97 Pike Street
Seattle, WA 98101
206-623-9837
essential oils, botanical products

Uncommon Herb
P.O. Box 2908
Seal Beach, CA 90740
800-845-0008
essential oils

Uncommon Scents
P.O. Box 1941
Eugene, OR 97440-1941
800-426-4336
fragrance oils, unscented shampoos

Zenith Supplies, Inc.
6300 Roosevelt Way N.E.
Seattle, WA 98115
206-525-7997
800-735-7217
essential oils, botanical products

INDEX